The System of Nature and the Balance of Life

Selections from Ibn Sīnā's Canon of Medicine

Ancient Wisdom Collection

Volume 1

About the Series

The Ancient Wisdom Collection
is devoted to translating, editing, and contextualizing the
foundational works of the world's great scientific and
philosophical traditions.

Each volume seeks to reintroduce classical knowledge as a
living intellectual system—not as relic or curiosity, but as a
coherent model of inquiry that continues to inform modern
thought.

Publisher's Preface

This volume inaugurates the *Ancient Wisdom Collection* with *The System of Nature and the Balance of Life*, selections drawn from *Ibn Sīnā's Canon of Medicine* (*al-Qānūn fī al-Ṭibb*).

The purpose of this translation is not merely to render the language of an ancient text into modern form, but to reveal the enduring logic of its system—a system in which the principles of life, matter, and balance cohere as one structure of knowledge.

Ibn Sīnā (Avicenna, 980–1037 CE) conceived medicine as the applied art of maintaining equilibrium within the living body. To him, the physician was both a scientist and a philosopher of nature, charged not only with healing disease but with understanding the laws that govern vitality itself.

This translation presents that vision anew—faithful to his terminology, rigorous in structure, and accessible to readers of medicine, philosophy, and the sciences alike.

Contents

Foundational Terms in the Canon of Medicine

In rendering Ibn Sīnā's *Canon*, several Arabic terms possess conceptual breadth that cannot be confined to a single English equivalent. Their meanings extend across physiology, philosophy, and metaphysics; thus, our translation will preserve their precision through a balance of English and selective transliteration.

The word *ṭibb* denotes not merely medicine as an applied craft, but a comprehensive *science of health*, encompassing the knowledge of the body's constitution, its preservation, and the restoration of balance when disturbed. Ibn Sīnā treats it as a rational discipline, governed by causes and demonstrable laws, rather than a mere accumulation of remedies.

Central to his physiology is the notion of *mizāj*, or temperament—the equilibrium arising from the blending of the four *arkān*, the primary elements of nature: fire, air, water, and earth. This balance of qualities—heat, cold, moisture, and dryness—determines the nature of bodies and the dispositions of living beings. We shall retain *mizāj* in transliteration, while rendering its meaning as "temperament" where context allows.

The elements themselves, *arkān* (singular *rukn*), will be translated as "elements," but when Ibn Sīnā employs them philosophically—as the fundamental components of corporeal existence—the Arabic form will occasionally be retained.

The *ṭabīʿa*, or "nature," is another central concept: it is the inner power or principle that directs each body toward its proper motion and function. It will generally appear in English as *nature*, though where Ibn Sīnā speaks of it as a specific physiological force—distinct from voluntary action—it may appear as *ṭabīʿa*.

The *quwā*—the "powers", "faculties", or "potential" of the body—comprise the vital, natural, and psychic functions by which life is maintained. This plural term (*quwā*, singular *quwwa*) will usually be rendered as "faculty" or "power," depending on the context: the *quwwa ḥayawāniyya* (vital faculty), *quwwa ṭabīʿiyya* (natural faculty), and *quwwa nafsāniyya* (psychic faculty).

Another fundamental pair of terms is *rūḥ* and *nafs*. The *rūḥ* (spirit) refers, in the medical sense, to the subtle substance generated in the heart and conveyed through the arteries as the carrier of life and sensation. The *nafs* (soul; self), though more philosophical, represents the principle of perception and movement, connected yet distinct from the corporeal *rūḥ*.

The term *qānūn*, meaning "law" or "canon," lends its title to the entire work. It signifies a system of universal principles that govern the art of medicine. In translation, it will appear as *Canon* when referring to the book itself, and as *law* or *universal rule* when used within the text.

When Ibn Sīnā speaks of *tashrīḥ*, he means anatomical exposition—the dissection and explanation of organs in relation to their functions (*manāfiʿ*). Both terms—*tashrīḥ* and *manfaʿa*—will be preserved in transliteration on first mention, followed thereafter by "anatomy" and "function."

The *a'ḍā'* (organs) are the structural members of the body, each possessing a purpose and composition suited to its role. The *a'ḍā' basīṭa* (simple organs) are the primary tissues such as bone, nerve, and muscle, while the *a'ḍā' murakkaba* (compound organs) are formed from them—like the hand, eye, or liver.

Ibn Sīnā's discussion of substances will distinguish between *adwiya mufrada* and *adwiya murakkaba*: simple and compound drugs. The first are natural substances used singly; the second are mixtures prepared according to specific ratios. For these, we will use "simple drug" and "compound drug," retaining *adwiya mufrada* and *adwiya murakkaba* only in the introductory passages of each section.

Finally, the term *aqrābādhīn* designates the pharmacopoeia—the collection of recipes, compounds, and methods of preparation. It was originally a Greek term (*grabadin*) adopted into Arabic medical literature. In the translation, *Aqrābādhīn* will be kept as a proper title for Ibn Sīnā's fifth book, and rendered as "Pharmacopoeia" in descriptive use.

Now...

Volume I — The Foundations of Natural Temperament and the Four Humors

(From Ibn Sīnā's Canon of Medicine, Ancient Wisdom Collection)

In this opening volume of Ibn Sīnā's monumental *Canon of Medicine*, the reader enters the living architecture of classical science—where health and disease are governed by balance, not chance. Here, the philosopher-physician unfolds the universal principles of life: the elemental roots of nature, the temperaments that shape bodies and dispositions, and the four humors—blood, phlegm, yellow bile, and black bile—through which vitality circulates and decline begins.

With clarity and precision, Ibn Sīnā reveals how moderation sustains existence and how its disturbance gives rise to illness. This first book thus forms the foundation of the entire medical art, offering both the logic and the ethics of care that unite body, soul, and cosmos.

The *Ancient Wisdom Collection* continues with the subsequent volumes of the *Canon*, each devoted to a distinct realm of knowledge—from the organs and their faculties, to the causes and cures of disease, and the composition of remedies—restoring to view one of humanity's most enduring systems of thought.

Book One

On the General Principles of the Science of Medicine

The first book on the universal principles of the science of medicine comprises four parts.

The first part concerns the definition of medicine and its subject matters among the natural sciences. It includes six teachings.

First Teaching

The first teaching consists of two sections.

Section One

I say: Medicine is a science through which one learns the conditions of the human body, viewed in respect to health and its loss, so that health may be preserved when it exists and restored when it has departed.

Someone may object and say that medicine is divided into theory and practice, yet you have made it entirely theoretical by defining it as a *science*. To such an objector we reply: Among the arts are those that are theoretical and those that are practical; and among the sciences of wisdom are also those that are theoretical and those that are practical. Likewise, in medicine there are aspects that are theoretical and others that are practical. However, the meaning of "theoretical" and "practical" is not the same in every context. It is not our present purpose to explain the difference in all cases, but only as it pertains to medicine.

When it is said that medicine is partly theoretical and partly practical, one should not suppose that this means the theoretical part belongs to knowledge alone while the practical part belongs solely to bodily action—as many who have examined this subject have mistakenly imagined. Rather, one must understand that the foundations of medicine are of two kinds: one is the knowledge of principles, and the other is the knowledge of the manner of their application. The first of these is properly called *science* or *theory*, and the second is called *practice*.

By *theory* in medicine we mean instruction that aims only at conviction and understanding, without concern for the manner of physical execution—such as when we say in medicine that fevers are of three kinds, or that temperaments are of nine. By *practice* we do not mean the manual or physical exercise itself, but that part of medical science whose instruction yields an opinion or judgment about *how* an act should be performed. For example, when it is said that in treating hot swellings one must first apply remedies that repel, cool, and resolve; then, after the initial stage, mix the cooling agents with softeners; and finally, when the inflammation subsides, restrict the treatment to softening and dissolving remedies—except in cases where the swelling arises from matter expelled by a principal organ—such an instruction provides a theoretical judgment regarding the manner of action.

Thus, when you have acquired both kinds of knowledge—the theoretical and the practical—you possess the complete science of medicine, even if you have never personally performed a treatment.

It should not be objected that the conditions of the human body are three—health, disease, and a third state that is neither health nor disease—whereas we have mentioned only two. For whoever reflects on this will find that neither the tripartition nor its omission is necessary. And even if such a tripartition were admitted, our statement that medicine concerns "the loss of health" already includes both disease and the intermediate state that is neither. For health is a disposition or condition by which the acts proper to the body are performed correctly. Whatever lacks this character stands as its contrary, whether or not it is a complete disease.

It is not our purpose to dispute with the physicians on this point; they are not accustomed to debate such matters, and such debates yield no benefit for medicine itself. The inquiry into the truth of these distinctions belongs rather to another art—the art of logic—and whoever desires that knowledge must seek it there.

Section Two

As for the *subject matters* of medicine: since medicine considers the human body in respect to its health and its loss, and since knowledge of anything is only complete when its causes are known, it follows that in medicine one must know the causes of health and disease. These causes, and the states they produce, may be evident to the senses or hidden, perceptible only by inference from their effects. Hence, medicine must also study those *symptoms* and *accidents* that occur in health and in disease.

It has been established in the demonstrative sciences that true knowledge of a thing arises through knowledge of its causes and its principles, when such exist; and when they do not, then through knowledge of its essential accidents and necessary attributes. The causes are of four kinds: material, efficient, formal, and final.

The *material causes* are the underlying substances in which health and disease subsist. The nearest of these subjects is the *organ* or the *spirit*; the more remote are the *humors*; and beyond these, the *elements* (*arkān*). These latter are subjects according to composition, though also according to transformation, for in every composition and transformation the multiplicity of parts tends toward some unity. That unity in this context is either a *mizāj* (temperament), in so far as it arises through transformation, or a *hay'a* (configuration), in so far as it arises through structure.

The *efficient causes* are those that change or preserve the conditions of the human body: the air and its qualities, foods, waters, and beverages, evacuation and retention, the regions and dwellings, bodily and psychic motions and rests—including sleep and wakefulness—the changes that occur with age, differences of species and occupations, habits, and whatever external factors come into contact with the body, whether agreeable to nature or contrary to it.

The *formal causes* are the temperaments, the faculties that arise from them, and the various compositions of the organs. The *final causes* are the actions themselves; and to know these actions necessarily requires knowledge of the *faculties* and of the *spirits* that bear them, as will be explained later.

These, then, are the subject matters of the medical art, insofar as it investigates the human body—how it remains healthy and how it falls ill. But from the standpoint of the perfection of this investigation, which is to preserve health and remove disease, medicine must also consider additional subjects corresponding to the causes and instruments of these two states. These include the management of diet and drink, the choice of air, the regulation of movement and rest, treatment by medicines, and treatment by hand.

All these matters, according to the physicians, pertain to three classes of people: the healthy, the sick, and those who are intermediate between the two. These intermediates we shall describe later, showing how they occupy a position between two states that in reality have no true middle.

Having thus set forth these distinctions, it becomes evident that medicine concerns itself with the elements, temperaments, humors, simple and compound organs, spirits and their natural, vital, and psychic faculties, with the actions of the body, and with the states of health, disease, and the intermediate conditions, together with their causes—foods, drinks, airs, waters, regions, dwellings, evacuations, retentions, occupations, habits, bodily and psychic movements and rests, ages, species, and external influences—and finally with the management of diet, drink, air, movement, and rest, and with therapy through drugs and manual operations, for the preservation of health and the treatment of disease.

Some of these things the physician must apprehend only in their *essence*—as scientific conceptions that he accepts as established by the natural philosopher. Others he must *demonstrate* within his own art. Whatever in medicine serves as a principle must be received as such; for the principles of the particular sciences are assumed and demonstrated in sciences more fundamental than themselves, until all finally ascend to *first philosophy*—that wisdom which is called *metaphysics*.

Thus, when some practitioners of medicine begin to speak of proving the existence of the elements or of temperament, or of other subjects that belong properly to natural philosophy, they err—first, because they introduce into medicine matters that do not belong to it, and second, because they imagine that they have demonstrated something when in truth they have not.

What the physician must apprehend as to *essence* and accept as established, though not self-evident, are these: that the elements exist, and how many they are; that the temperaments exist, what they are, and how many; that the humors exist, what they are, and how many; that the faculties exist, and how many; that the spirits exist, how many they are, and where they reside; and that every change and every permanence has a cause, and that the causes are of four kinds.

As for the organs and their uses, these must be perceived by sense and through *tashrīḥ* (anatomy). What the physician must both apprehend and demonstrate are the particular diseases, their specific causes and signs, and the manner by which disease is removed and health preserved. In such matters he must provide demonstration for whatever is obscure in its existence—through analysis, estimation, and confirmation.

Galen, when he sought to demonstrate matters belonging to the first class, did so not as a physician but as a philosopher concerned with natural science. Similarly, when a jurist endeavors to prove the obligation of following consensus, he does not do so as a jurist but as a theologian engaged in speculative reasoning. The physician, *qua* physician, and the jurist, *qua* jurist, cannot prove such principles directly; if they attempt it, they fall into circular reasoning.

The Second Teaching

On the Elements (*al-arkān*)

It consists of one section.

The elements are simple bodies, primary parts of the human body and of other beings. They are those bodies that cannot be divided into parts differing in form, and into which compounds are ultimately resolved. By their blending there arise the various species of forms among generated things. The physician should receive from the natural philosopher that they are four and only four: two are light and two are heavy. The light ones are fire and air; the heavy ones are water and earth.

Earth is a simple body whose natural place is at the center of the whole. There, by nature, it remains at rest; and to that place it naturally moves, if set apart from it. This is its absolute heaviness. Its natural quality is cold and dry; that is, its nature—left to itself and to what it requires, without any external cause altering it—manifests sensible coldness and dryness. Its presence among generated things confers firmness, stability, and the preservation of shapes and configurations.

Water is a simple body whose natural place is to encompass the earth while being encompassed by the air, when earth and air occupy their proper natural positions. This is its relative heaviness. Its natural quality is cold and moist; that is, its nature—left to itself and to what it requires, without an opposing external cause—exhibits sensible cold and the condition called moisture. Moisture means that in its constitution it responds to the slightest cause by separating and reuniting, receiving any shape, then not preserving it. Its role among generated things is to allow the succession of configurations wherever shaping, outlining, and adjustment are desired. For though the moist readily abandons imposed shapes, it readily receives them; and though the dry is resistant to receiving shapes, it is resistant to abandoning them. Whenever the dry is leavened with the moist, the dry gains from the moist an easy capacity for extension and shaping; and the moist gains from the dry a strong capacity to preserve whatever rectification and adjustment have occurred. Thus the dry is gathered from dispersion by the moist, and the moist is held back from flowing by the dry.

Air is a simple body whose natural place is above water and beneath fire. This is its relative lightness. Its natural quality is hot and moist, according to the measure already explained. Its role among generated things is to loosen, subtilize, lighten, and enable elevation.

Fire is a simple body whose natural place is above all the elemental bodies. Its proper place is the concave surface of the celestial sphere at which generation and corruption cease. This is its absolute lightness. Its natural quality is hot and dry. Its function among generated things is to ripen, subtilize, and blend, and to run through them by opening pathways in the airy substance; it moderates the sheer cold of the two heavy, cold elements, so that they turn back from the state of mere elementality to a *temperamental* state. The heavy elements are more helpful in the constitution of organs and in their rest; the light elements are more helpful in the constitution of the *spirits* and in their motion and in moving the organs—though the first mover is the *soul*, by the permission of its Creator. These, then, are the elements.

The Third Teaching

On the Temperaments (*al-amzija*)

It consists of three sections.

Section One

On temperament

I say: Temperament (*mizāj*) is a quality arising when contrary qualities interact and then come to a stand at a certain limit. It occurs when the elements, reduced to very small parts so that each touches more of the others, interact by their powers, each in the other, and from their total there emerges a quality that is uniform throughout—this is temperament. The primary powers in the aforesaid elements are four: heat, cold, moisture, and dryness. The temperaments found in generated and corruptible bodies arise from these, and reasoned division, considered absolutely and without relation to any subject, shows two principal ways of conceiving them.

One way supposes a perfectly *moderate* temperament, in which the measures of the contrary qualities in the mixture are equal and counterpoised, and temperament would then be a quality precisely intermediate among them. The second way does not make temperament an absolute middle between the contraries, but makes it inclined toward one of the sides, either in one of the contrary pairs—heat versus cold, or moisture versus dryness—or in both pairs.

Yet what counts in the medical art regarding moderation and deviation from it is not either of these conceptions. The physician must accept from the natural philosopher that moderation in that first strict sense cannot exist at all—let alone be the temperament of a human being or of a human organ. He must know that the *moderate* employed by physicians in their discussions is derived not from equality as exact balance, but from *equity* in due apportionment: namely, that the compound—whether a whole body or a single organ—has received, from the elements in their quantities and qualities, the share fitting for it in the human temperament according to the most just division and proportion. It may happen that this apportionment approaches very closely the first, true moderation; and this moderation, considered with respect to human bodies, is also relative—by comparison to other beings that do not possess such moderation, not by proximity to the impossibility mentioned earlier.

A person's nearness to that supposed strict moderation can be considered under eight regards. It may be considered, first, by species, in comparison to what lies outside that species; or, second, by species in comparison to what differs within it. Third, by a class within the species, compared to what lies outside it and within its own kind; or, fourth, by that class compared to what differs within it. Fifth, by an individual of a given class and species, compared to what lies outside, within the class, and within the species; or, sixth, by that individual compared to the differences of his own states across time. Seventh, by an organ, compared to what lies outside it and within the body; or, eighth, by that organ compared to its own states.

The first of these is the moderation that belongs to the human being in comparison with the rest of generated things. This has breadth and is not confined within a single fixed limit, yet it is not without measure; it has bounds of excess and deficiency, and when one departs beyond them the temperament ceases to be a human temperament. The second is the mean between the two extremes of that broad human temperament; it occurs in an individual at the height of moderation, belonging to a class likewise at the height of moderation, at the age when growth reaches its perfection. Although this is not the strict, impossible moderation described at the beginning of the section, it is nonetheless difficult to find. Such a person approaches true moderation not by chance, but because his organs that are hot, such as the heart, and those that are cold, such as the brain, and those that are moist, such as the liver, and those that are dry, such as the bones, are balanced and counterpoised; when they are thus balanced, they approach true moderation. Considered organ by organ—save for one, namely the skin, as will be described—this may hold. But with respect to the *spirits* and the principal organs, it cannot be close to the strict moderation; rather, it must incline toward heat and moisture. For the principle of life is the heart and the spirit, and both are very hot and tend toward excess; life depends on heat, and growth on moisture; indeed, heat is sustained by moisture and is nourished by it. The principal organs are three, as will be explained; among them only one is cold, the brain, and its cold does not suffice to counterbalance the heat of the heart and the liver. Only one is dry, or nearest to dryness, namely the heart, and its dryness does not suffice to counterbalance the moist temperament of the brain and the liver. Nor is the brain so extremely cold, nor the heart so extremely dry; but in relation to the others, the heart counts as dry and the brain as cold.

The third consideration is narrower in breadth than the first (the species-wide moderation), though it still has a fair latitude. It is the temperament suitable for a given *nation* by comparison with a given *climate* and air. Thus India has a temperament in which its inhabitants remain healthy; the Slavs have another temperament in which they remain healthy; each is moderate relative to its own class and not moderate relative to the other. When a body of Indian constitution is altered to the Slavic temperament, it falls ill or perishes; likewise, a Slavic body altered to the Indian temperament fares the same. Each group of the earth's inhabitants therefore has its own temperament appropriate to the air of its clime. The fourth consideration is the mean within the range of a given climate's temperament; this is the most moderate temperament for that class.

The fifth is narrower than the first and the third. It is the temperament that an individual must have in order to exist as a living, healthy person. This also has a latitude bounded by two limits, excess and deficiency; and you should know that every person deserves a temperament proper to himself, which rarely—or perhaps never—another shares with him. The sixth is the mean between those two limits for that same person; when it is realized, he is in the best state befitting him.

The seventh is the temperament required for the kind of each organ, by which it differs from other organs. Thus the moderation proper to bone is that dryness predominates in it; for the brain, that moisture predominates; for the heart, that heat predominates; and for nerve, that cold predominates. This organ-kind moderation also has a latitude bounded by excess and deficiency, narrower than the latitudes mentioned for the temperaments above. The eighth is the moderation specific to each individual organ, by which the organ is in the best possible condition of its own temperament; it is the mean between the two limits and, when realized, sets the organ in its optimal state.

If you consider species, the one nearest to true moderation is the human being. If you consider the classes within humanity, it has been established with us that, provided the region along the equinoctial line is inhabited and no terrestrial factors oppose—such as mountains and seas—its inhabitants should be the class nearest to true moderation. The opinion that departs from this on the ground of the sun's nearness is unsound; for the sun's direct culmination there causes less injury and alteration of the air than its oblique approach here at greater latitudes without culmination. Moreover, all their other conditions are excellent and uniform; the air does not conflict with them in a markedly perceptible way, and their temperament is consistently similar. We once composed a treatise to confirm this view. After these, the most moderate of the classes are the inhabitants of the fourth clime: they are neither scorched by the sun's frequent culmination over their heads, as in much of the second and third climes, nor chilled by its constant remoteness, as in much of the fifth and higher latitudes.

As for individuals, the most moderate is the most moderate person of the most moderate class of the most moderate species. As for the organs, it has appeared that the principal organs are not very close to true moderation; you should know that flesh is among the organs nearest to that moderation, and nearer still is the skin. The skin is scarcely affected by water mixed in equal parts—half frozen and half boiling—and the warming from the vessels and blood is nearly balanced by the cooling from the nerves. Likewise it is not affected by a well-mixed substance composed equally of the driest and the most fluid bodies. We know it is unaffected because it does not perceive: if it were contrary to it, it would be affected by it, for things of common element but opposite natures act upon one another; a thing fails to be affected only when what acts shares with it a similarity in the relevant quality. The most moderate skin is that of the hand; of the hand, the palm; of the palm, that which is upon the fingers; of the fingers, that which is upon the forefinger; and of that, the skin upon its last phalanx. For this reason, it and the tips of the other fingers are almost the judge by touch in measuring tangible qualities, since the judge should be equally inclined to both extremes, so as to sense when either extreme departs from the middle and from equity.

you should also understand—together with what has already been explained—that when we say of a drug that it is *moderate*, we do not mean that it is moderate *in the strict sense*, for that is impossible; nor do we mean that it is moderate by the *human* standard of temperament, for then it would share the very substance of the human body. Rather, we mean that when the drug is affected by the innate heat (*al-ḥarāra al-gharīziyya*) in the human body and takes on a certain quality thereby, that acquired quality does not depart from the human quality toward either extreme beyond due balance; hence it exerts no effect that bends away from moderation. In this way, it is *as if* moderate with respect to its action in the human body. Likewise, when we call a drug *hot* or *cold*, we do not mean that in its essence it is at the utmost degree of heat or cold, nor that its essence is hotter or colder than the human body; otherwise, what we called moderate would simply be that whose temperament is identical to the human. We mean only that from the drug there arises in the human body a heat or a cold exceeding what the body already possesses. For this reason, a drug may be cold with respect to the human body yet hot with respect to the body of a scorpion; and hot with respect to the human body yet cold with respect to the body of a snake. Indeed, one and the same drug may act as hotter upon the body of Zayd than it does upon the body of ʿAmr. Hence practitioners are instructed not to persist with a single drug when attempting to alter a temperament if it does not avail.

Having completed the account of the moderate temperament, let us turn to the non-moderate. Whether you take them in relation to the species, the class, the individual, or the organ, the non-moderate temperaments are eight, all opposed to the moderate. They arise in the following way. Departure from moderation may be *simple*, occurring in one contrariety only, or *compound*, occurring in both contrarieties. The simple departure in a *primary* (active) contrariety is twofold: either hotter than is fitting—without being moister or drier than is fitting—or colder than is fitting—without being drier or moister than is fitting. The simple departure in a *secondary* (passive) contrariety is likewise twofold: either drier than is fitting—without being hotter or colder than is fitting—or moister than is fitting—without being hotter or colder than is fitting.

These four do not remain fixed for any considerable time. What is hotter than is fitting soon makes the body drier than is fitting; what is colder than is fitting makes the body moister than is fitting—by an alien moisture. What is drier than is fitting quickly renders it colder than is fitting; and what is moister than is fitting—if in excess—cools it even more swiftly than dryness does; but if not excessive, it preserves it somewhat longer, yet in the end leaves it colder than is fitting. From this you may understand that *moderation*—or health—is more consonant with *heat* than with *cold*. These, then, are the four simple departures.

As for the *compound* departures, in which the excess involves both contrarieties, they are such as: hotter *and* moister together than is fitting; or colder *and* moister together than is fitting; or colder *and* drier together than is fitting. It is not possible for something to be hotter and colder together, nor moister and drier together.

Each of these eight temperaments may occur either *without matter* or *with matter*. Without matter: the temperament arises in the body as a mere quality, without the body's being altered by the penetration of a humor qualified by that temperament—such as the heat of a part that has been vigorously pounded or the cold of loins numbed and frozen. With matter: the body's change of temperament is due to the presence of a humor penetrating and prevailing in it—such as the cooling of the human body by *vitreous phlegm* (*balgham zujājī*), or its heating by a *leek-like yellow bile* (*ṣafrāʾ kurrāthī*). In the third and fourth books you will find an example for each one of the sixteen temperaments thus distinguished.

Know also that temperament *with matter* occurs in two ways. Sometimes the organ is permeated by the matter and *imbued* with it; and sometimes the matter is retained in its channels and cavities. Its retention and insinuation may produce a swelling, or it may not.

Section Two

On the Temperaments of the Organs

Know that the Creator—exalted and glorified be He—has bestowed upon every living being, and upon each organ within it, the temperament most fitting and most beneficial for its actions and functions, according to what is possible for it. The demonstration of this belongs properly to the philosopher rather than to the physician. The human being has been granted the most balanced temperament attainable in this world, suited to the powers by which he acts and is acted upon. Likewise, every organ has been endowed with the temperament appropriate to it: some of the organs are hotter, others colder; some drier, others moister.

The hottest of all within the body is the *spirit* and the *heart*, its origin and source. Next comes the *blood*, for although it is generated in the liver, by its connection to the heart it acquires a degree of heat that the liver itself does not possess. After these, the *liver* follows, being itself a coagulated form of blood. Then come the *lungs*, then the *flesh*, which is somewhat cooler owing to the admixture of the cold nerve fibers. After flesh comes *muscle*, cooler than the simple flesh because of its mixture with nerve and ligament; then the *spleen*, due to the turbidity of the blood it contains; then the *kidneys*, since the blood there is not abundant. Next in order are the coats of the *arteries that pulse*, not because of their fibrous substance but because of the heat imparted by the blood and spirit within them; then the coats of the *veins that do not pulse*, heated only by the blood; and after these, the *skin of the palm*, which is of a moderate temperature.

The coldest substance in the body is *phlegm*, followed by *fat*, then *hair*, then *bone*, then *cartilage*, then *ligament*. The moistened order is the opposite. The moistest of all bodily substances is *phlegm*, then *blood*, then *fatty tissue*, then *adipose fat*, then *the brain*, then *the marrow*, then *the flesh of the breast and the testes*, then *the lungs*, then *the liver*, then *the spleen*, then *the kidneys*, then *muscle*, and finally *skin*. This is the arrangement recorded by Galen.

But one must understand that the lungs, in their essence and innate disposition, are not extremely moist; for every organ's natural temperament resembles that of the substance from which it is nourished, and its accidental temperament resembles that of what it excretes. The lungs are nourished by the hottest blood and the most mingled with yellow bile. Galen himself teaches this; but it also happens that the lungs accumulate much accidental moisture, both from the vapors rising through the body and from the descending discharges that flow into them.

If this is the case, then the *liver* is much moister than the lungs in its innate moisture, while the lungs are more subject to wetness by exposure and persistence of dampness, which may even render their very substance moister. In this way you should also understand the relation between *phlegm* and *blood*: the moisture of phlegm is, for the most part, *superficial and adhesive*, whereas the moisture of blood is *substantial and cohesive*. The natural, watery phlegm may be, in itself, more moist; for when blood reaches its due ripeness, much of the moisture that existed in the natural watery phlegm from which it was transformed departs from it. You will later learn that natural phlegm is blood that has undergone only a partial transformation.

The driest substance in the body is *hair*, for it is formed from a smoky vapor whose moisture has been dissipated and whose dry, sooty part has condensed. Next comes *bone*, which is the hardest of the organs; it is harder than hair, because bone originates from blood and is so situated as to absorb and master the innate moisture. For this reason, bone serves as nourishment for many animals, whereas hair does not nourish at all, or does so rarely, as has been supposed in the case of bats, which are thought to digest it. Yet if we take equal weights of bone and hair, and distill them together in an alembic, more water and oil will flow from the bone, and it will leave a lighter residue. Thus bone is in truth moister than hair.

After bone in dryness comes *cartilage*, then *ligament*, then *tendon*, then *membrane*, then *artery*, then *vein*, then *motor nerve*, then *heart*, and finally *sensory nerve*. The motor nerve is both colder and drier than the moderate mean; the sensory nerve is colder, but not much drier than the mean—perhaps indeed near to it, and not far removed even in its coldness. After these comes *skin*.

Section Three

On the Temperaments of the Ages and of the Sexes

The ages of life are, in general, four. The first is the *age of growth*, also called the *age of youthfulness*, extending to nearly thirty years. The second is the *age of steadiness*, the age of *maturity or full youth*, continuing to about thirty-five or forty years. The third is the *age of decline while strength remains*, the age of the *middle-aged*, lasting to about sixty years. The fourth is the *age of decline with manifest weakness*, the age of *old age*, which continues to the end of life.

The age of growth itself is divided into several stages. The first is *infancy*, when the newborn's organs are not yet ready for movement or rising. The next is *childhood*, between rising and firmness, when the teeth have not yet completed their falling and replacement. Then comes *early adolescence*, following firmness and the complete growth of the teeth but before puberty. After that is the *age of boyhood and approaching maturity*, until facial hair begins to sprout. Finally comes *the age of the youth*, which continues until growth ceases.

Children—that is, from infancy until early youth—have a temperament that is moderate in *heat* and excessive in *moisture*. The ancient physicians differed regarding the relative heat of the child and the young man. Some held that the child's natural heat is stronger, since his growth is greater, his natural functions—desire, digestion, and the like—are more active and enduring, because the innate heat derived from the semen is more abundant and fresher.

28

Others held that the heat of young men is much stronger, because their blood is more plentiful and robust; hence they are more subject to nosebleeds, and their temperament inclines more toward yellow bile (*ṣafrā'*), whereas that of children inclines toward phlegm (*balgham*). Their movements are stronger, and movement itself arises from heat; their digestion and assimilation are also stronger, and these likewise come from heat.

As for *sexual desire*, it does not arise from heat but from coldness; for this reason, rabid lust most often originates from cold temperaments. The proof that the young are better at digestion is that they are less prone than children to nausea, vomiting, and indigestion, which come from poor digestion. The proof that their temperament leans more toward yellow bile is that their diseases are all hot—such as tertian fevers—and their vomit is bilious; whereas most diseases of children are moist and cold, their fevers phlegmatic, and their vomit largely phlegmatic.

Growth in children, then, is not due to the strength of their heat but to the abundance of their moisture; likewise, the excess of appetite in them indicates a deficiency of heat. Such are the opinions and arguments of both parties.

Galen, however, refuted both, holding that the heat in both children and youths is equal in origin, but differs in quantity and quality: the heat of children is greater in *quantity* yet lesser in *quality* (that is, in sharpness), whereas the heat of youths is lesser in *quantity* yet greater in *quality* (that is, in intensity). To explain this, he imagined one and the same heat, equal in amount and degree, diffused now in a very moist substance like water, and again in a very dry substance like stone. In the first case, the hot water would be greater in quantity but gentler in quality; in the second, the hot stone would be smaller in quantity but sharper in quality. So it is with the heat in children and in youths. Children are generated from the semen, itself full of heat; that heat has not yet been diminished by any extinguishing cause. The child is still advancing in increase and growth and has not yet reached his limit—how, then, could his heat be receding?

The youth, on the other hand, has neither a cause to augment his innate heat nor yet one to extinguish it; that heat remains conserved in him, but with a lesser measure of moisture both in quantity and quality, until the beginning of decline. The reduction of this moisture is not small in relation to the preservation of heat, but only in relation to growth. At first, moisture suffices for both preservation and increase; later, it suffices for preservation but not for increase; at last, it suffices for neither. Therefore, in the middle period, it suffices for one—preservation—but not the other—growth. It is impossible to say that it would suffice for growth but not for preserving innate heat; for how could that which cannot preserve its cause increase beyond it? It follows, then, that moisture suffices to preserve innate heat but not to promote growth—and this stage is the age of youth.

As for the claim that growth in children arises only from moisture and not from heat, it is false; for moisture is only the *material* of growth, and matter does not shape or act upon itself but only under the action of a formative power. The acting power here is the soul or nature, by God's permission, and it acts only through an instrument—namely, innate heat. Similarly, their claim that the strong appetite of children arises from coldness of temperament is false, for that disordered appetite which comes from coldness is not accompanied by proper digestion and assimilation. Children, however, in most cases digest in the best manner; otherwise they could not absorb from their food more than they lose, as they must do in order to grow.

It is true, however, that they may suffer indigestion through greed, poor discipline in eating, the consumption of bad, moist, or excessive foods, and through untimely or disordered movements. Hence, they accumulate more excess matter and need more frequent purification—especially in the lungs. Their pulse is therefore more frequent and rapid, though not strong, for their strength is not yet complete.

This, then, is the account of the temperament of the child and the youth, following Galen's exposition as we have rendered it. You must also know that after the period of steadiness, heat begins to decline, because the surrounding air dries up its material, which is moisture; and this is aided by the innate heat within and by bodily and psychic movements necessary for living, while nature is unable to resist indefinitely. All bodily powers are finite; hence their actions of replenishment cannot continue without limit. Were they infinite and constant, replenishment and loss would remain equal; but since loss is not equal and increases daily, the replacement cannot keep pace. Dissolution consumes the moisture; and when both forces—dissolution and deficient replacement—conspire toward decrease, it necessarily follows that the material is exhausted and the heat extinguished, especially as extinction is hastened by another cause: the foreign moisture that arises continually through imperfect digestion, smothering and opposing the innate heat.

Such is *natural death*, allotted to each person according to his temperament; to each a fixed term and a written limit, differing from one to another by the diversity of temperaments. These are the *natural terms* of life, whereas there are also *accidental* deaths of another kind, each likewise determined in measure.

The result of all this is that the bodies of children and youths are moderately warm, while those of adults and the aged are cold. Yet the bodies of children are moister than the mean, because of growth—shown by the softness of their bones and nerves—and this agrees with both experience and reasoning, for they are still near in origin to the semen and to the vaporous spirit. Adults and especially the aged are, on the contrary, not only colder but drier, as experience shows in the hardness of their bones and the dryness of their skin, and as reason shows from their distance in time from the seminal substance, blood, and vaporous spirit.

The fiery element is equal in children and youths; the airy and watery are greater in children; the earthy greater in adults and the aged, and greatest in the aged. The youth's temperament is more balanced than the child's— dry relative to him, but hot relative to the man of middle or old age. The old man is drier than both youth and adult in his essential organs, but moister than they in extraneous, corrupt moisture.

As for *the sexes*, their temperaments differ likewise. Women are colder than men, and therefore smaller in stature and less perfect in formation; they are also moister, so that because of their cold temperament their superfluities are more abundant, and because of their lesser exercise, the substance of their flesh is looser. The flesh of men, though looser in texture because of its mixture with sinew and vessel, is by its density cooler than what pervades the flesh of women.

In the same way, *the inhabitants of northern lands* are moister, as are those whose livelihoods depend upon water; their opposites are the drier. The signs of these temperaments will be described later, when we speak of the general and particular indications.

The Fourth Teaching

On the Humors

It consists of two sections.

Section One

The nature of humor and its kinds

A humor is a moist, flowing substance into which food is first transformed. Of humors, some are *commendable*: these are of such a sort as to become part of the very substance of the nourished body—either by themselves or together with others—and to resemble that substance—either by themselves or together with others—so that, in sum, they replace something of what has been dissolved and lost. Others are *bad humors*: these are not of such a sort, or they are transformed into the commendable humor only rarely; their proper course, before that, is to be repelled from and purged out of the body.

We accordingly say: the body's moistures are either *primary* or *secondary*. The primary moistures are the four humors that we are about to describe. The secondary moistures are of two kinds: either *superfluities* (which we shall mention later) or *non-superfluities*. By the latter we mean moistures that have passed out of their initial state and have penetrated the organs but have not yet become, in act and in full perfection, the very substance of any simple organ. These are of four sorts:

34

(1) The moisture confined within the cavities at the extremities of the vessels;

(2) The moisture diffused through the principal organs like dew—ready to be converted into nourishment when the body lacks incoming food, and ready to moisten organs that have been dried by violent movement or other causes;

(3) The moisture *recently coagulated*, namely the nourishment that has been transformed toward the substance of the organs by way of *temperamental assimilation* and likeness, though not yet transformed by way of complete consistency;
(4) The moisture that has been *interwoven* with the principal organs from the very beginning of growth, by which their parts cohere—its origin is from the semen (*nutfa*), and the origin of the semen is from the humors.

We also say: both the commendable humoral moistures and the superfluous moistures are contained under four genera—blood, which is the noblest; phlegm; yellow bile; and black bile.

Blood is hot and moist by nature. It is of two kinds: *natural* and *unnatural*. Natural blood is red in color, not fetid, and distinctly sweet. Unnatural blood is of two sorts. In one, the temperament itself has departed from its proper balance, not by admixture with anything foreign but by alteration within itself—becoming, for example, colder or hotter than it ought. In the other, the alteration arises from the admixture of a *bad humor*; this, again, is of two kinds: either a foreign humor has entered from outside and penetrated the blood, corrupting it; or the humor has arisen within the blood itself—so that one portion has putrefied and turned a thin layer into yellow bile, pungent and bitter, or into thick black bile, and one or both remain mingled with it. This second kind, with its two modes, varies according to what mingles with it—types of phlegm, of black bile, of yellow bile, or of watery fluid—so that sometimes the blood becomes turbid, sometimes thin, sometimes very black, sometimes whitish; likewise its odor and taste alter—becoming bitter, salty, or tending toward sourness.

Phlegm is also of two kinds, natural and unnatural. *Natural phlegm* is that which is apt, at some time, to become blood, for it is blood not yet fully matured; it is a kind of sweet phlegm. It is not intensely cold: with respect to the body it is mildly cold; with respect to blood and yellow bile it is cold. There is also a sweet phlegm that is *not* natural: this is the tasteless phlegm that we shall mention when it happens to be mixed with natural blood, often perceived in catarrhs and in expectoration.

As for the *sweet natural phlegm*, Galen claims that nature has not assigned to it a specific excretory organ, as it has for the two bitters, because this phlegm is near in kind to blood and all the organs need it; therefore it is conducted along the same course as the blood. We say: that need is of two kinds—one a *necessity*, the other a *benefit*. The necessity is for two reasons. First, that it may be near to the organs, so that whenever they lack the incoming nourishment—whether because the supply from the stomach and liver is cut off, or for some incidental reasons—their faculties turn to it with the innate heat, cook and digest it, and are nourished by it. Just as innate heat ripens, digests, and rectifies it into blood, so also an *accidental heat* corrupts and putrefies it. This necessary function is not shared by

36

the two bitters (yellow and black bile); for they do not share with phlegm the property that innate heat renders it blood—though they do share with it that accidental heat can make it putrid.

Second, natural phlegm mingles with the blood and prepares it to nourish organs of *phlegmatic temperament* which require that their nutritive blood contain *actual phlegm* in a determinate proportion—for example, the brain. This function the bitters also possess.

The *benefit* of natural phlegm is that it moistens the joints and the organs of frequent motion, so that they do not dry out from movement and friction. This benefit, indeed, approaches the level of necessity.

Unnatural phlegm includes superfluous varieties that differ in consistency even to sense: this is the *mucous* kind. It also includes varieties that seem uniform to sense yet differ in reality: this is the *raw* phlegm. Among its kinds is the very *thin, watery* phlegm; and the very *thick, white* phlegm called *gypsum-like*, which has separated into layers from being long retained in joints and passages—this is the thickest of them all. There is also a *salty phlegm*, which is the warmest, driest, and most desiccative among the phlegms.

Every saltness arises when a watery moisture of little or no taste is mixed with earthy particles that have been *burned*—dry in temperament and bitter to the taste—in due proportion; if those earthy parts are excessive, the result becomes bitter. From this process, salts are generated and waters become saline. Salt, moreover, may be made from ash, *qali* (alkali), *nūra* (natron/lime), and the like: by boiling them in water, straining, and then evaporating the water until it congeals into salt—or simply by leaving it until it congeals. In just this way, thin, tasteless—or but faintly flavored—phlegm, when moderately mixed with a naturally dry, combust, bitter substance, becomes saline and heated: this is *bilious phlegm* (phlegm tinged with the property of yellow bile).

The excellent sage Galen has said that such phlegm becomes salty because of *putrefaction* or because *wateriness* has mixed with it. We say: putrefaction makes it saline by inducing in it a kind of burning and ashiness that commingles with its moisture. But the mere admixture of watery fluid does not by itself produce saltness unless the second cause is present as well.

There is also a *sour phlegm*. Just as sweetness may be of two sorts—one from a property in the thing itself, the other from an alien admixture—so too sourness is twofold: one arises from mixing with some foreign thing, namely the *sour black bile* that we shall describe; the other arises from a property in the phlegm itself, as when the sweet phlegm described above—or that which is tending toward sweetness—undergoes, like other sweet juices, *ebullition* first and *acidification* thereafter.

There is further an *astringent* phlegm (*'afṣ*). Sometimes its astringency is due to admixture with astringent *black bile*; at other times it occurs because the phlegm itself has become intensely cold in its essence, so that its taste turns astringent when its watery part hardens and inclines toward earthiness. In such a case, weak heat is insufficient to boil it into sourness, while strong heat is lacking to ripen it into perfection.

Among the types of *phlegm* there is one that is *glassy*—thick and heavy, resembling molten glass in its viscosity and weight. It is sometimes *sour* and sometimes *insipid*. The thick insipid kind seems to be the *raw phlegm*, or what becomes raw phlegm through transformation. This form of phlegm was originally *watery* and *cold*; it neither putrefied nor mingled with any other substance but remained confined until it thickened and grew colder.

From this, it is clear that the *corrupted phlegms* are of four kinds by *taste—salty, sour, astringent,* and *insipid*—and of four kinds by *consistency—watery, glassy, mucous,* and *gypsum-like*. The *raw phlegm* lies in preparation between the mucous and the glassy kinds.

As for *yellow bile (ṣafrā')*, it too is of two kinds: *natural* and *unnatural*. The natural kind is the *foam of the blood*—bright red, light, and sharp. The hotter it is, the redder it becomes. When it is generated in the liver, it divides into two portions: one passes with the blood, the other is strained off into the gallbladder.

That which goes with the blood does so by *necessity* and *benefit*. Necessity, because it must mix with the blood to nourish organs that require in their temperament some portion of yellow bile in due proportion—such as the lungs. Benefit, because it *thins* the blood and helps it *penetrate narrow channels*.

That which is separated and carried to the *gallbladder* also serves necessity and benefit. Necessity, either for the *body as a whole*, in that it purges excess, or for the *gallbladder itself*, which it nourishes. Benefit, likewise, is twofold: one, that it *washes the intestines* of fecal matter and viscous phlegm; the other, that by its acrid sting it stimulates the intestines and the muscles of the rectum to perceive the need for evacuation and to prompt defecation. This is why sometimes *colic* arises.

The *unnatural* yellow bile is either *abnormal by admixture with a foreign substance* or *abnormal in its own essence*. The first kind is more common and well known—it is that in which the foreign admixture is *phlegm*, and it usually arises in the *liver*. There is also a less common form, where the foreign admixture is *black bile*. The well-known forms are of two types: the *pure yellow bile (murrat ṣafrā')* and the *milky bile (murrat muḥiyya)*. When the phlegm that mingles with it is thin, the first kind results; when it is thick, the second kind arises—the bile resembling the *white of an egg*.

The less common kind is called *burnt yellow bile (ṣafrā' muḥtariqa)*. It appears in two ways: first, when the yellow bile itself burns, acquiring a grayish hue in which the fine and the ashen parts are mingled and inseparable—this is the *worst* and most harmful form. The second occurs when *black bile* comes upon it from without and mixes with it— this is less harmful. The color of this burnt type is reddish, but dull and clouded, resembling blood though thinner, and it may vary in color according to circumstance.

As for the yellow bile that is abnormal *in its essence*, part of it is generated mainly in the *liver*, and part mainly in the *stomach*. The one produced in the liver is a single kind—the *fine portion of blood when burned*, leaving behind its thick residue as *black bile*. The kinds formed in the stomach are two: *leek-green (kurrāthī)* and *verdigris-like (zanjārī)*.

The *leek-green bile* seems to arise from the burning of the *milky bile*, for when the latter burns, the combustion produces blackness that mixes with the yellowness, yielding a greenish hue between the two. The *verdigris-like bile* arises, it seems, from the further burning of the leek-green kind, when its moisture has been exhausted and its color turns whitish from excessive dryness. For heat first produces *blackness* in a moist body, then, when it consumes the moisture, *whitens* it. Consider wood: first it becomes charcoal, then ashes. Heat thus darkens moisture and whitens its opposite; cold likewise whitens moisture and blackens its opposite.

These accounts of the leek-green and verdigris-like bile are conjectural, yet the *verdigris type* is the *hottest, most noxious, and most deadly* of all yellow biles. It is said to share the nature of *poisonous substances*.

As for *black bile (sawdā')*, it also has *natural* and *unnatural* forms. The natural kind is the *residue and sediment of good blood*, thick and turbid, its taste between sweetness and astringency. When it forms in the liver, it divides into two parts: one goes with the blood, the other toward the spleen.

The part that goes with the blood does so by necessity and benefit. Necessity, so that a proper measure of black bile mixes with the blood to nourish organs requiring it in their temperament—such as *bones*. Benefit, in that it *strengthens, thickens, and stabilizes* the blood, preventing its rapid dissipation.

The part that goes to the *spleen*, being the portion superfluous to the blood, goes also for necessity and benefit.

Necessity, for the body as a whole, is *purification from excess*; for the spleen itself, it is *nutrition*. Benefit arises when it *flows back to the mouth of the stomach* after its transformation; this, too, has two effects: it *fortifies and thickens the stomach's mouth*, and by its *acidity it tickles it*, awakening hunger and stimulating appetite.

Know that the bile that drains into the gallbladder is that which the blood no longer needs, and that which drains out from the gallbladder is what the gallbladder no longer requires. Likewise, the black bile that drains into the spleen is what the blood no longer needs, and that which drains out of the spleen is what the spleen no longer requires. Just as the yellow bile that leaves the gallbladder stimulates the *expulsive faculty* from below, so this black bile that leaves the spleen stimulates the *attractive faculty* from above. Blessed is God, the best of creators and the wisest of judges.

The *unnatural black bile* is not formed by sedimentation and settling but by *burning and ashen transformation*. Moist substances mixed with earthiness differentiate their earthy part in two ways: either by *settling*—as in the natural black bile, the dregs of the blood—or by *burning*, where the fine part is consumed and the thick remains, as in burnt residue. This second kind, occurring in blood and humors, is the *unnatural black bile*, also called *the burnt bile (murrat sawdā')*.

Sedimentation occurs only in blood, because phlegm, being viscous, does not settle like dregs, and yellow bile, being subtle, light, and ever moving, has too little earthy substance to settle. When separated, it quickly putrefies or is expelled, and in putrefying, its fine part vanishes while its coarse part remains as *burnt, not sedimentary, black bile.*

Among these *unnatural black biles*, some are the *ashes and burnings of yellow bile*, which are *bitter*; the difference between these and the *burnt yellow bile* is that in the latter the ash is mixed with the bile, while here the ash is separated and independent. Others are the *ashes of phlegm*; if the phlegm was very fine and watery, its ash inclines toward *saltness*; otherwise it inclines toward *sourness* or *astringency*. Others are the *ashes of blood*, which are *salty with a touch of sweetness*. Others still are the *ashes of natural black bile*: if it was thin, its ash and burning are intensely *acid*, like *vinegar boiling upon the earth*, with a pungent smell that repels flies; if thick, it is less acid, tinged with *astringency and bitterness.*

Thus the *corrupt kinds of black bile* are three: (1) yellow bile when burnt and its fine part consumed; (2) the two subsequent forms just described—the ashes of bile and of other humors.

The *phlegmatic black bile*—that which arises from the burning of phlegm—is the *slowest in harm* and the *least noxious* of them all.

These four humors, when subjected to burning, are ranked in wickedness. *Black bile* is the worst and most baleful; *yellow bile* spoils the quickest, yet is the most amenable to treatment. As for the other two, that which is *most acid* is the worse; however, if it is met promptly at its outset, it is more tractable to cure. The *third* (by which is meant the less effervescent upon the ground, less adherent to the organs, and slower to bring about destruction) is longer in reaching its fatal end.

Galen spoke rightly, and those erred who claimed that the only *natural* humor is blood, while all the others are merely superfluities that are never needed. Were blood alone the humor that nourishes the organs, their temperaments and consistencies would be all alike. Bone would not be harder than flesh unless the blood that nourishes it were mingled with a *black, earthy* principle; the brain would not be softer unless its blood were mingled with a *soft, phlegmatic* principle. Indeed, you will find blood itself mixed with the other humors: when it is drawn and allowed to settle in a vessel under the witness of sense, it separates into a froth resembling yellow bile, a portion like the white of egg resembling phlegm, a sediment and turbidity resembling black bile, and a watery portion—the *aqueous*—whose excess is driven off in the urine. The aqueous is not counted among the humors, for it comes from drink, which does not nourish; it is needed only to *thin the nourishment and conduct it*. A humor, by contrast, comes from the food and the nutritive drink; by *nutritive* we mean that which is potentially similar to the body. What is potentially like the human body is a *mixed* substance, not a simple one; water is simple.

Some suppose that the body's strength depends on the *quantity* of blood, and its weakness on the paucity of it. Not so: what matters is the *condition* of the body's share of blood—that is, the *goodness* of its state. Others suppose that if the humors, after having once been in the proportions that the human body requires relative to one another, increase or decrease while preserving those relative proportions, health is preserved. Not so: each humor must also keep a due *absolute measure* in itself—not merely in proportion to another humor—while also preserving its relational measure. There remain inquiries concerning the humors that it does not befit physicians to pursue, for they belong not to our craft but to the philosophers; therefore we pass them over.

Section Two: On the manner in which the humors are generated

Know that food undergoes a first digestion by *mastication*. This is because the surface of the mouth is continuous with the surface of the stomach—indeed, as if they were one surface—and the mouth possesses a digestive force. When the chewed morsel comes into contact with it, the mouth effects a certain alteration in it, aided by the *saliva*, itself made fit by the ripening that arises in it from innate heat. Hence it is that *chewed wheat* ripens boils and abscesses in a way that wheat merely pounded with water or boiled in it does not. They say: the evidence that the chewed morsel has begun to ripen is that its first taste and first odor are no longer found in it.

When the morsel arrives at the stomach, it is completely digested—not by the stomach's heat alone, but also by the heat of what *surrounds* it: on the right, the *liver*; on the left, the *spleen*, which is warmed not by its own substance but by the many arteries and veins within it; in front, the *omentum* laden with fat, which quickly receives heat because of the fat that conveys it to the stomach; and from above, the *heart*, which transmits warmth through the diaphragm. Once digested at first, the food becomes—of itself in many animals, and with the help of the drink mixed with it in most—*chyle*: a flowing substance like thick barley water or the milky water of *kashk*, smooth and white.

Thereafter its *subtle portion* is drawn from the stomach—and from the intestines as well—and is carried along the *mesenteric loop* (the *mesaraic* veins), which are fine, firm vessels attached to the whole length of the intestines. From there it passes into the *portal vein* of the liver and penetrates the liver through its many small branches, narrow like hairs, meeting the mouths of the roots of the *ascending* vessel that issues from the liver's convexity. Because it passes through these narrow channels, the chyle—mixed with a portion of potable water, more than the body itself requires—spreads through the fibers of these vessels so that the entire liver, as it were, is in contact with the entire chyle; the liver's action upon it is thus stronger and quicker. Then it *cooks*, and in every such cooking there arises something like *froth* and something like *dregs*; sometimes there is also a portion tending toward *burning* if the cooking exceeds due measure, or toward *rawness* if the cooking falls short.

The froth is *yellow bile*; the dregs are *black bile*—both *natural*. Of what is burnt, the subtle becomes *bad yellow bile*, and the thick becomes *bad black bile*—both *unnatural*. What is *raw* is *phlegm*. The well-cooked, well-clarified portion is *blood*. Yet while it remains in the liver, the blood is *thinner* than it should be, because of the surplus watery portion required for the reason just mentioned; but as soon as it departs from the liver, it is further *clarified* of that superfluous water which was needed only for a time, and this water is drawn off through a *descending vessel* to the *kidneys*. With it goes that part of the blood, in quantity and quality, that suits the nourishment of the kidneys, which are fed by the fatty and sanguine part of that water; the rest is driven into the *bladder* and out through the *urethra*.

The well-constituted blood, meanwhile, ascends through the vessel arising from the liver's convexity, courses through the branching veins, then through their *rivulets*, then their *channels*, then their *lateral feeders*, then the *hair-like fibrous vessels*; from their mouths it *transudes* into the organs—*in the measure decreed by the Mighty, the All-Knowing*. Thus the *efficient cause* of blood is *moderate heat*; its *material cause* is the *moderate, choice foods and drinks*; its *formal cause* is *excellent ripening*; and its *final cause* is the *nutrition of the body*.

The efficient cause of *yellow bile* is, for the *natural* (the blood's froth), *moderate heat*; for the *burnt* form, *excessive, fiery heat*—especially in the liver. Its material cause is *fine, hot, sweet, fatty,* and *pungent* foods; its formal cause is *overpassing ripeness into excess*; its final cause is the *necessity and benefit* previously described.

The efficient cause of *phlegm* is *deficient heat*; its material cause is *thick, moist, viscid, cold* foods; its formal cause is *imperfect ripening*; its final cause is its *necessity and benefit* as set forth before.

The efficient cause of *black bile* is, for the *sedimentary* kind, *moderate heat*; for the *burnt* kind, *excessive, immoderate heat*. Its material cause is *very thick foods of little moisture*; among hot foods, those that are intense are strong in producing it. Its formal cause is *dregs that settle* in such a way as either *not to flow* or *not to dissolve*; its final cause is its *necessity and benefit* as mentioned. Black bile increases through *heat of the liver, weakness of the spleen, intense freezing cold, persistent retention,* or *many and prolonged illnesses* that have *scorched* the humors. When black bile abounds and *stagnates between the stomach and the liver,* the generation of blood and of good humors diminishes, and *blood is reduced.*

You must also know that *heat* and *cold* are causes of humoral generation together with the other causes. *Moderate heat* generates *blood; excessive heat* generates *yellow bile; very excessive heat,* by *over-burning,* generates *black bile. Cold* generates *phlegm; very great cold,* by *over-freezing,* generates *black bile.* Yet one must also consider the *passive capacities* of the recipient in relation to the *active powers;* it is not necessary to believe that every temperament always produces its like and produces its opposite only accidentally and never essentially. Often a temperament *produces its opposite:* a *cold, dry* temperament produces *alien moisture,* not by likeness, but because of *weak digestion.* Such a person is slender, with lax joints, timorous, cold to the touch and smooth-skinned, with narrow vessels. Similarly, *old age* produces *phlegm,* though the temperament of old age is truly *cold and dry.*

Know further that the *blood and what courses with it in the vessels* undergo a *third digestion;* and when distributed to the organs, each organ performs a *fourth digestion.* The residue of the *first digestion* (in the stomach) is expelled by way of the intestines. The residue of the *second digestion* (in the liver) is discharged mostly in the urine, and the rest by way of the spleen and the gallbladder. The residues of the *third and fourth digestions* are carried off by *insensible perspiration,* by *sweat,* and by *scurf* that exits partly through sensible outlets (the nose and ear canal) or insensible ones (the pores), or by *unnatural exits* such as *ruptured swellings*, or by what *grows from the body as excrescences*—hair and nail.

Know that the *thinner the humors*, the *weaker their evacuation*, and the more the person is harmed by *wide pores*, because the weakness that follows dissolution injures the strength; thin humors are easy to evacuate and dissolve, and what is easily evacuated and dissolved easily carries off the *spirit* with it in dissolution, so that the spirit *dissolves along with it*. And as these humors have causes for their *generation*, so too they have causes for their *motion*: *movement* and *hot things* stir the *blood* and *yellow bile*, and sometimes *move and strengthen black bile*; whereas *repose* strengthens *phlegm* and certain kinds of *black bile*. Even *imaginations* move the humors: *blood* is stirred by looking upon *red things*; thus the person with nosebleed is forbidden to gaze upon objects that glitter red.

This is what we have to say concerning the humors and their generation; as for disputations with opponents about the truth of these matters, that belongs to the philosophers rather than to physicians.

Commentary

The System of Nature and the Principle of Balance in Ibn Sīnā's Medical Philosophy

In the opening book of *The Canon of Medicine*, Ibn Sīnā constructs not merely a manual of healing, but a science of life in its most comprehensive sense. What appears at first as an exposition of elements, temperaments, and humors unfolds into a profound philosophy of balance—an explanation of how the human body participates in the universal order of nature. Every statement in this book, from the structure of the organs to the qualities of heat and cold, belongs to a system whose purpose is to understand *how being persists through equilibrium and perishes through excess.*

The Architecture of Balance

For Ibn Sīnā, medicine begins where philosophy leaves off: at the point where the principles of natural bodies become principles of living bodies. He inherits from the ancients—Aristotle, Galen, and Hippocrates—the conviction that the universe is composed of simple elements whose mixtures give rise to all forms. Yet he surpasses them in method and clarity.

In his treatment of *mizāj* (temperament), he converts the static notion of mixture into a dynamic law of proportion. Heat, cold, moisture, and dryness are not substances but relational forces; health itself is the state of their mutual moderation. Disease, therefore, is not an invasion from without but a deviation within—a systemic failure of equilibrium.

This vision is strikingly modern. Where contemporary biology speaks of *homeostasis, metabolic regulation*, and *adaptive response*, Ibn Sīnā spoke of *moderation of temperament*—the same self-correcting intelligence of nature that sustains life. The vocabulary differs, but the conceptual architecture is identical: living systems endure only through continual adjustment to preserve their inner ratios.

The Four Humors as Systemic Media

In the second half of this book, Ibn Sīnā develops the classical doctrine of the *four humors*—blood, phlegm, yellow bile, and black bile—not as inert fluids but as *functional media of transformation*. Each humor represents a phase of the body's material process: generation, nourishment, and decay. The humors are, in effect, the *circulating expressions of temperament*.

Modern readers, trained in chemical physiology, may find this taxonomy archaic. Yet a closer reading reveals an astonishing anticipation of systemic biochemistry. Blood as the warm, vital medium; phlegm as the nutritive reserve and regulator of hydration; yellow bile as the agent of metabolic heat and excretion; and black bile as the stabilizer of structure and density—these correspond to observable physiological domains that remain intelligible even in molecular terms. Ibn Sīnā's error, if one may call it that, is not in principle but in vocabulary. He described processes by their qualities rather than by their molecules; the underlying logic remains valid.

More importantly, his analysis of humoral transformation—how food becomes blood, blood becomes tissue, and waste becomes fuel or poison—is essentially a theory of metabolism, centuries before the term existed. It conceives the body not as a vessel of fluids but as a *continuum of change.* In this sense, Ibn Sīnā's medicine is more holistic and systematic than much of modern practice, which often isolates mechanisms but loses sight of the system's unity.

Knowledge as *Integration*

The *Canon* thus teaches that the art of medicine is inseparable from the science of nature and the ethics of proportion. Health is not the absence of illness but the continuity of right relation: between elements in the body, between the body and its environment, between human reason and the intelligence of the cosmos. The physician's task is not only to treat disease but to understand *how the order of nature expresses itself in the human frame.*

This insight explains why Ibn Sīnā's medicine endured for nearly a millennium as the dominant scientific paradigm across civilizations—from Andalusia to Persia, from Latin Europe to India. It persisted because it was more than empirical; it was *systemic.* It drew upon the collective wisdom of earlier civilizations—Greek, Persian, Indian, and Islamic—synthesizing them into a rational and moral science. Its method was integrative before the term existed.

Relevance for the Modern Sciences

To students of medicine and the biological sciences today, *Book I* (not to be confused with *Volume 1, our serialized translation of the entire work*) remains not an artifact but a mirror. It reminds us that the human organism is not a machine to be repaired but a system to be understood in its natural and ethical totality. It invites us to restore to medicine its philosophical depth—to see in every diagnostic value and cellular process a reflection of the same law of balance that Ibn Sīnā called *mizāj*.

As this series continues, the reader will see how the same systemic vision unfolds across all domains of life: from the structure and function of organs, to the operations of the faculties, to the causes and cures of disease. Each subsequent book will build upon the foundation established here—where matter becomes life through equilibrium, and knowledge becomes healing through understanding.

In recovering Ibn Sīnā's *Canon*, we are not returning to the past. We are retrieving the lost continuity of knowledge—the wisdom that recognized no boundary between physics and ethics, between the science of the body and the harmony of the world.

Publisher's Note

The Foundations of Natural Temperament and the Four Humors

This first volume of *The Canon of Medicine* introduces the fundamental architecture of Ibn Sīnā's medical philosophy—his vision of the human body as a balanced system governed by elemental qualities, temperamental moderation, and the interplay of the four humors. In these teachings, the physician is not merely a healer of disease but a student of equilibrium itself: understanding how heat, cold, moisture, and dryness combine to generate the living order, and how their excess or deficiency gives rise to disorder.

Through these chapters, the reader encounters the framework upon which classical medicine was built: the logic of *mizāj* (temperament), the differentiated constitution of the organs, the cycles of human life, and the great doctrine of the *akhlāt*—blood, phlegm, yellow bile, and black bile—which together sustain the material and vital processes of the body. The reflections that close this section—on the generation of the humors, their causes, transformations, and moral significance—mark the end of Ibn Sīnā's general physics of health, and the threshold of his physiology of action.

The forthcoming volumes in this *Ancient Wisdom Collection* will continue the journey into the deeper structures of the Canon. *Volume 2* will explore the organs, faculties, and vital spirits that execute nature's design; *Volume 3* will treat the diseases of specific organs and their therapies;

Volume 4 will examine systemic ailments and the care of beauty; and *Volume 5* will complete the work with the study of compound remedies.

With the completion of *Volume 1*, the reader stands at the gateway of Avicenna's medical cosmos—a world where body, soul, and nature are joined by the same laws of proportion and purpose.

Appendices

Appendix I

Intellectual Lineage and Referenced Authorities

Ibn Sīnā's *Canon of Medicine* stands at the summit of a thousand years of inquiry into life, balance, and the human body. It is not an isolated achievement, but a culmination— a conscious act of synthesis that unified the scattered insights of Greek, Hellenistic, and early Islamic medicine into a single, coherent science. To know its lineage is to perceive the *Canon* not merely as a medical manual, but as a monumental philosophy of health.

The Greek Foundations

Hippocrates (Buqrāṭ) laid the conceptual cornerstone with the doctrine of humors: that health arises from equilibrium (*i'tidāl*) among the four fluids—blood, phlegm, yellow bile, and black bile—and that disease is their disequilibrium. Ibn Sīnā preserved this structure but grounded it in a richer causal framework linking physiology, temperament, and cosmic order.

Galen (Jālīnūs) refined Hippocratic doctrine through anatomy and logic. Ibn Sīnā revered Galen's precision yet distinguished observation from speculation, subjecting each Galenic assertion to systematic reason. He re-anchored medicine in purpose: every organ exists for a teleological end, every motion for a function within a balanced whole.

Aristotle (Arisṭūṭālīs) supplied the metaphysical logic. From the Aristotelian four causes, Ibn Sīnā drew the model of medical explanation: *material* (the body's substance), *formal* (its organization), *efficient* (its active power), and *final* (its purpose). Thus, health became not a mechanical condition but a harmony of intention and matter.

Dioscorides and other Greek pharmacologists enriched Ibn Sīnā's materia medica. He absorbed their empirical catalogues but reclassified each substance by its systemic effect on human *mizāj*, transforming lists of drugs into a theory of balanced interaction.

Late-Classical and Alexandrian Contributors

Rufus of Ephesus, Paul of Aegina, and the physicians of Alexandria transmitted Hellenic medicine through Syriac intermediaries. Their anatomical lexicon reached Ibn Sīnā, who extended it by ordering all bodily functions within a hierarchy of systems—the natural (*ṭabī ʿī*), the vital (*ḥayawānī*), and the psychic (*nafsānī*).

Islamic Synthesis and Critical Innovation

Among his Muslim predecessors, *al-Rāzī (Rhazes)* emphasized clinical observation and contagion, while *al-Fārābī* built the philosophical architecture reconciling Aristotle and Plato. Ibn Sīnā absorbed both legacies: empiricism from the former, structural rationalism from the latter. He merged Greek science with Qurʾānic cosmology, creating a medicine that served body and soul alike.

Through this synthesis, the *Canon* became more than a compendium of cures; it became an epistemology of health—a vision where reason and nature converge. The physician, in Ibn Sīnā's view, is not a technician but a guardian of equilibrium, charged with maintaining the correspondence between the human microcosm and the cosmic macrocosm.

Thus the *Canon of Medicine* represents civilization's maturity: the meeting of observation, logic, and moral purpose. Its endurance across centuries reminds the modern student that medicine's ultimate aim is not domination over nature, but understanding and participation in its balance.

Appendix II

The System of Health According to Ibn Sīnā

(A conceptual map rendered in descriptive form, faithful to his medical philosophy and aligned with systems thinking.)

Ibn Sīnā envisioned the human organism as *a self-regulating system* mirroring the structure of the cosmos. Life endures through the measured interplay of heat and cold, moisture and dryness—forces that continuously negotiate the state of equilibrium called health.

1. The Elements (*Arkān*) — Foundations of Existence

All material beings arise from four elemental natures:

Element	Primary Qualities	Symbolic Role
Air	hot & moist	mediation, vitality
Fire	hot & dry	transformation, motion
Water	cold & moist	cohesion, nourishment
Earth	cold & dry	solidity, stability

These qualities combine in infinite ratios, producing the diversity of bodies and dispositions.

2. The Temperament (*Mizāj*) — Law of Balance

From elemental mixture arises *mizāj*, the composite temperament that defines each body's natural constitution.

- Perfect balance yields health.

- Deviation produces vulnerability or disease.

Each organ bears a temperament fitted to its work: the heart warm and subtle, the brain cool and moist, the liver temperate and nutritive. Human diversity of character and resilience stems from differences in these proportions.

3. The Humors (*Akhlaṭ*) — Vehicles of Life

Nutrition generates four circulating substances that mediate vitality:

1. Blood (*dam*) — warm & moist; life-giving, red, nourishing.

2. Phlegm (*balgham*) — cold & moist; lubricating, softening.

3. Yellow bile (*ṣafrā'*) — warm & dry; stimulating, cleansing.

4. Black bile (*sawdā'*) — cold & dry; stabilizing, consolidating.

Health requires purity and proportionality among them; disorder in kind or quantity leads to pathology.

4. The Faculties (*Quwā*) — Engines of Vital Function

Three interlocking faculties sustain organic life:

- Natural faculty (*quwwa ṭabī'iyya*) — nutrition, growth, reproduction.

- Vital faculty (*quwwa ḥayawāniyya*) — pulse, circulation, animation.

- Psychic faculty (*quwwa nafsāniyya*) — perception, imagination, voluntary motion.

Each faculty depends upon the others; together they compose the living equilibrium.

5. The Role of the Physician

The physician restores balance by discerning which quality—heat, cold, dryness, or moisture—has departed from moderation. Therapy, whether by regimen, diet, or compound medication, acts through contraries: the cold is warmed, the dry moistened, the moist dried, the hot cooled. Healing is thus *systemic correction*, not symptomatic suppression.

6. The Systemic Cycle

From a systems-theory perspective, Ibn Sīnā's model forms a dynamic feedback loop:

Elements → Temperament → Humors → Faculties → Functions → Re-balancing of Temperament

Disturbance at any level affects all others. Environmental forces—climate, food, emotion—enter this circuit; the physician intervenes to restore adaptive stability. Disease appears when regulation fails; recovery is the re-establishment of harmonious feedback.

7. Enduring Insight

To Ibn Sīnā, the human body is a microcosm of ordered motion. Health is not stasis but the rhythmic maintenance of proportion within change. His *Canon* anticipates modern ecological and systemic medicine by portraying life as a self-organizing equilibrium rather than a mechanical assembly.

The lesson endures: *to heal is to cooperate with nature's design*, not to command it. The physician's art, the philosopher's wisdom, and the theologian's awe converge upon the same truth—that balance is the law of being.

Glossary of Key Terms

On the Elements, Temperaments, and Humors

(All transliterations follow a modified ALA–LC standard; technical definitions are rendered in modern, accessible English while preserving Avicennian precision.)

A

'Adam al-tawāzun (عدم التوازن) — *imbalance*; the disruption of equilibrium among the elemental qualities (heat, cold, moisture, dryness), leading to illness or dysfunction.

A'ḍā' (أعضاء) — *organs*; the functional components of the body, each possessing a distinct *mizāj* suited to its operation.

Akhlāṭ (أخلاط) — *humors*; the four fundamental bodily fluids — blood (*dam*), phlegm (*balgham*), yellow bile (*ṣafrā'*), and black bile (*sawdā'*) — whose balance maintains health and whose excess or deficiency causes disease.

Asbāb (أسباب) — *causes*; in Avicenna's system, the efficient, material, formal, and final principles determining physiological processes.

B

Balgham (بلغم) — *phlegm*; the cold and moist humor. When balanced, it supports lubrication, nourishment, and calm temperament; in excess, it causes lethargy, coldness, and congestion.

Barūdah (برودة) — *coldness*; one of the four elemental qualities, counteracting *ḥarārah* (heat). It contracts, congeals, and stabilizes substances.

D

Dam (دم) — *blood*; the hot and moist humor, considered the most balanced and nourishing. It sustains vitality and growth, providing warmth and movement to the body.

Dardī al-dam (دردي الدم) — *residue of blood*; the coarse, dense portion of blood that settles as *sawdā'*, responsible for strength and structure.

F

Fa'il (فاعل) — *active cause*; in physiology, the agent that acts upon matter — for instance, the innate heat in digestion.

Fasād (فساد) — *corruption*; the degradation of a humor or temperament from its natural state, often by excess heat, cold, or putrefaction.

G

Ghalaba (غلبة) — *dominance*; when one quality or humor predominates, causing an imbalance (*ghalabat al-ṭabī'ah*).

Ghidhā' (غذاء) — *nourishment*; food and drink that, through digestion and transformation, become part of the body's substance.

H

Ḥarārah (حرارة) — *heat*; the active, vital principle that animates life, associated with expansion, motion, and transformation.

Ḥumrā' (حمراء) — *redness*; the natural hue of *dam*, signifying purity and vitality in humoral balance.

Ḥumūm (حموم) — *burnt residues*; carbonized remains resulting from excessive heat during digestion, often producing corrupt humors like *sawdā' muḥtariqah* (burnt black bile).

K

Kabid (كبد) — *liver*; the central organ of humoral production, where food is transformed into *dam* and its derivatives (*ṣafrā', balgham, sawdā'*).

Kayfiyyah (كيفية) — *quality*; refers to the qualitative attributes (hot/cold, moist/dry) that determine a body's temperament.

Kaylūs (كيلوس) — *chyme*; the semi-fluid substance formed in the stomach before its conversion into blood within the liver.

M

Mā'iyyah (مائية) — *watery essence*; the liquid component in the humors or the body, responsible for fluidity and solvency.

Mizāj (مزاج) — *temperament* or *mixture*; the balanced blending of the four elemental qualities in a body or organ. Ibn Sīnā defines *mizāj* as the *equilibrium of interaction between opposing qualities*, giving each organ its natural constitution.

Muḥtariqah (محترقة) — *burnt*; applied to humors altered by excessive heat or combustion, e.g., *ṣafrā' muḥtariqah* (burnt bile).

Mizāj al-insān (مزاج الإنسان) — *the human temperament*; the most balanced form of *mizāj* found in nature, enabling both physical and intellectual perfection.

N

Nafs ṭabī'iyyah (نفس طبيعية) — *the natural soul*; the vital principle directing the body's growth, nourishment, and reproduction — distinct from the rational soul.

Nudj (نضج) — *maturation* or *concoction*; the process by which crude matter (e.g., food, humors) is ripened by innate heat until it reaches functional perfection.

Nukha' (نخاع) — *marrow*; the moist substance within bones, associated with *balgham* and vital lubrication.

Q

Qiwā (قوى) — *faculties*; the powers or capacities through which the soul acts in the body — natural, vital, and psychic.

Qūwah ṭabī'iyyah (قوة طبيعية) — *natural faculty*; the power responsible for nutrition, growth, and reproduction.

Qūwah ghādhiyah (قوة غاذية) — *nutritive faculty*; the specific function of transforming food into bodily substance.

R

Rūḥ (روح) — *spirit*; the subtle, vaporous essence arising from the most refined blood, serving as the medium of the soul's actions in the body. It is the seat of vital heat.

Rūṭūbah (رطوبة) — *moisture*; one of the elemental qualities, enabling flexibility, union, and nourishment.

S

Ṣafrā' (صفراء) — *yellow bile*; the hot and dry humor, facilitating digestion and movement. In excess, it causes inflammation, irritability, and heat-related disorders.

Ṣafā' (صفاء) — *purity*; the refined and balanced state of a humor, free of corruption.

Sawdā' (سوداء) — *black bile*; the cold and dry humor, the sediment of blood. It provides structure and stability but in excess produces melancholy and obstruction.

Sūdāwī (سوداوي) — *melancholic*; a temperament dominated by *sawdā'*.

T

Ṭabī'ah (طبيعة) — *nature*; the inherent organizing power that directs bodily functions toward equilibrium and preservation.

Tadbīr (تدبير) — *regimen* or *management*; the art of maintaining or restoring balance through diet, exercise, and environment.

Takhalluf (تخلّف) — *residual accumulation*; leftover matter that fails to transform completely, often becoming a source of disease.

Takhallul (تخلّل) — *permeation*; the process of humors diffusing through tissues and vessels.

Tarkīb (تركيب) — *composition*; the structural combination of elements and qualities forming a natural body.

Tawāzun (توازن) — *equilibrium*; the balance among the four qualities and humors that defines health.

Z

Zanjārī (زنجاري) — *verdigris-like bile*; a highly corrosive form of *ṣafrā'*, resembling copper rust in color, produced by extreme heat and associated with toxic states.

Zujājī (زجاجي) — *vitreous phlegm*; a thick, glassy, gelatinous form of *balgham*, caused by cold constriction and lack of transformation.